HEALT RECIPES FOR BEGINNERS

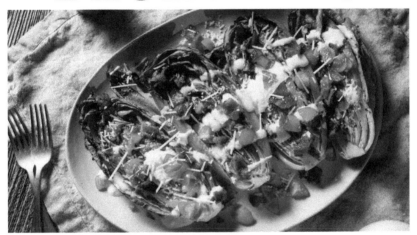

SIDES

Paola Clifford

Welcome!

To this new series of book, inspired by all the recipes I know thanks to my great passion: *cooking!*

"You really know what you are eating if you make it yourself"

In this book you will find many different ideas for your dishes, with ingredients from all around the world, with a Gourmet touch!

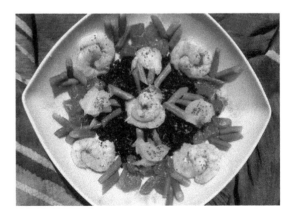

Thanks to these cookbooks you can develop your cooking skills for any kind of meal, as you'll find recipes for:

- ★ salads
- ★ sides
- ★ lunch
- ★ dinner
- ★ Desserts

And much more...

Whether your favourite dish is French fries, muffins, chicken tenders or grilled vegetables, with this series of books you will learn how to do it with a better-looking touch!

Don't forget that this books have also low fat recipes with healthy ingredients to *keep you fit and have a healthier meal plan!*

Remember that having a wide variety of ingredients and foods in your diet have many benefits for you, that's why you will find ingredients from:

- ★ Asia
- ★ Russia
- ★ America
- ★ Europe

And much more...

Since I started to pay more attention on the decision of the ingredients and how to plate a dish, I enjoy cooking a lot more! That's why I made this cookbook for all of you that want to develop your cooking skills and start eating healthier!

 I hope you will enjoy this book! Don't forget to check out the other ones from the collection, and enjoy your time in the kitchen!

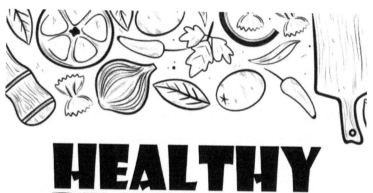

HEALTHY RECIPES
FOR BEGINNERS

SIDES

LEARN HOW TO MIX DIFFERENT INGREDIENTS AND SPICES TO
CREATE DELICIOUS DISHES AND BUILD A COMPLETE MEAL PLAN!
THI COOKBOOK INCLUDES QUICK RECIPES TO PREPARE ON A
DAILY BASIS, FOR AN EFFECTIVE DIET AND A HEALTHIER LIFESTYLE!

Paola Clifford

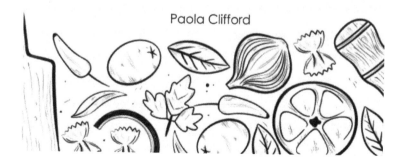

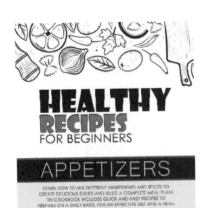

HEALTHY RECIPES FOR BEGINNERS: APPETIZERS

Learn how to mix different ingredients and spices to create delicious dishes and build a complete meal plan! This cookbook includes quick recipes to prepare on a daily basis, for an effective diet and a healthier lifestyle!

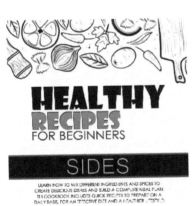
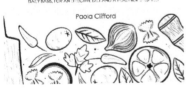

HEALTHY RECIPES FOR BEGINNERS: SIDES

Learn how to mix different ingredients and spices to create delicious dishes and build a complete meal plan! This cookbook includes quick recipes to prepare on a daily basis, for an effective diet and a healthier lifestyle!

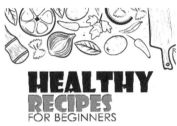

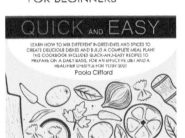

HEALTHY RECIPES FOR BEGINNERS: QUICK AND EASY

Learn how to mix different ingredients and spices to create delicious dishes and build a complete meal plan! This cookbook includes quick-and-easy recipes to prepare on a daily basis, for an effective diet and a Healthier lifestyle for your 2021!

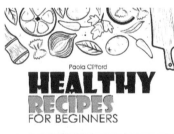

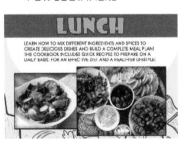

HEALTHY RECIPES FOR BEGINNERS: LUNCH

Learn how to mix different ingredients and spices to create delicious dishes and build a complete meal plan! This cookbook includes quick recipes to prepare on a daily basis, for an effective diet and a healthier lifestyle!

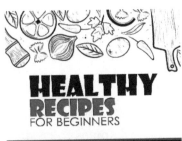

HEALTHY RECIPES FOR BEGINNERS: DESSERTS

Learn how to mix different ingredients and fruit to create delicious desserts and build a complete meal plan! This cookbook includes quick and easy recipes for both adults and kids, from the Mediterranean and other well-

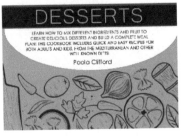

known diets!

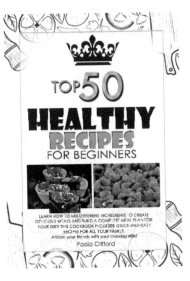

HEALTHY RECIPES FOR BEGINNERS: TOP 50

Learn how to mix different ingredients to create Delicious meals and build a complete meal plan for your diet! This cookbook includes quick-and-easy recipes for all your family. Amaze your friends with your cooking skills!

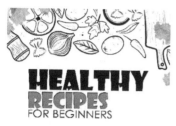

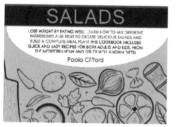

HEALTHY RECIPES FOR BEGINNERS: SALADS

Lose weight by eating well! Learn how to mix different ingredients and fruit to create delicious salads and build a complete meal plan! This cookbook includes quick and easy recipes for both adults and kids, from the mediterranean and other well-known diets!

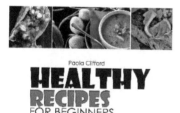

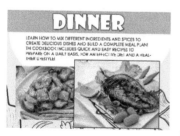

HEALTHY RECIPES FOR BEGINNERS: DINNER

Learn how to mix different ingredients and spices to create delicious dishes and build a complete meal plan! This cookbook includes quick and easy recipes to prepare on a daily basis, for an effective diet and a healthier lifestyle!

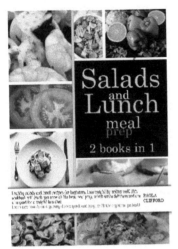

SALADS AND LUNCH MEAL PREP

2 books in 1: Healthy salad and lunch recipes for beginners. Lose weight by eating well! This cookbook contains some of the best low-fat recipes that also ideal for weight loss and body-healing routines. Improve your cooking skills with the right book!

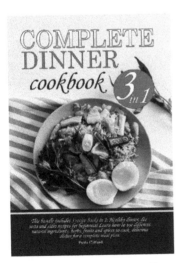

COMPLETE DINNER COOKBOOK

This boundle contains 3 recipe books in 1: healthy dinner, desserts and sides recipes for beginner.

Learn how to use different ingredients, herbs, spices and plants to cook delicious dishes for your complete meal plan.

Table of Contents

THE MAIN SIDES FOR YOUR MEALS

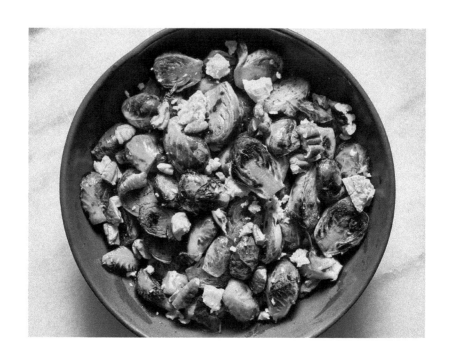

Fettuccini Tomato Rustica

Serving: 4

Ingredients

- 1 cup olive oil

- 2 cloves garlic, chopped

- 10 sun-dried tomatoes, chopped

- 1 roasted red pepper, diced

- 2 teaspoons dried basil

- 8 ounces dry fettuccini noodles

- 4 grilled skinless, boneless chicken breast halves

- 1/2 cup crumbled goat cheese

Direction

- Mix basil, red pepper, sun-dried tomatoes, garlic and olive oil in a small bowl. Allow to marinate for 4 hours.

- Preheat the oven to 120°C or 250°F. Boil a big pot of lightly salted water. Put pasta; let cook till al dente or for 8 to 10 minutes. Allow to drain. Toss the pasta along with marinade till equally coated. Scatter into a baking dish.

- In preheated oven, bake for an hour. Distribute among plates, put grilled chicken on top, and drizzle goat cheese over.

Nutrition Information

- Calories: 970 calories;

- Total Carbohydrate: 46.2

- Cholesterol: 96

- Protein: 42.6

- Total Fat: 69

- Sodium: 369

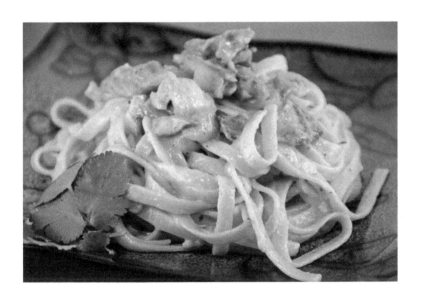

Finocchi Al Gratin (Fennel Gratin)

Serving: 4

Ingredients

- 2 tablespoons bread crumbs, or as needed

- 2 bulbs fennel bulbs, cut into wedges

- 3 tablespoons butter

- 1/3 cup all-purpose flour

- 1 1/2 cups milk

- 3 tablespoons milk

- salt and ground black pepper to taste

- 1 pinch ground nutmeg

- 2 tablespoons grated Parmesan cheese

Direction

- Preheat an oven to 175 °C or 350 °F. Grease a baking dish and scatter bread crumbs over the dish.

- In a saucepan, put a steamer insert and fill with water to just under the bottom of steamer. Boil. Put in fennel wedges, cover, and steam for 10 minutes till soft yet crisp. Drain and put into a baking dish.

- In a big skillet, melt butter over medium heat. Mix in flour to create a soft paste. Slowly beat in 1 1/2 cups plus 3 tablespoons of milk; simmer for 5 to 6 minutes till sauce is thick and creamy. Put in nutmeg, pepper and salt to season.

- In the baking dish, spread sauce on top of fennel. Scatter Parmesan cheese over the top.

- In the prepped oven, bake for 20 minutes till golden. Broil for 2 to 3 minutes till top is browned. Let sit for 5 minutes prior to serving.

Nutrition Information

- Calories: 227 calories;

- Total Fat: 12

- Sodium: 266

- Total Carbohydrate: 23.9

- Cholesterol: 33

- Protein: 7.4

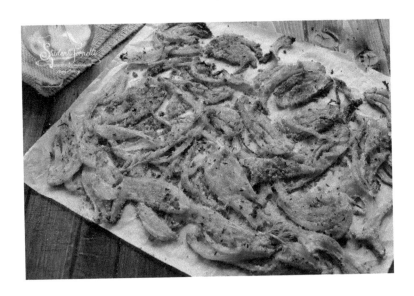

Fried Green Beans

Serving: 4

Ingredients

- 2 tablespoons extra virgin olive oil

- 1 tablespoon butter

- 2 tablespoons fresh lemon juice

- 2 cups diagonally sliced fresh green beans

- 1 teaspoon lemon zest

- 1 pinch garlic salt to taste

- 1 pinch ground black pepper to taste

Direction

- In a skillet over medium-high heat, heat the lemon juice, butter and olive oil.

- Put in pepper, garlic salt, lemon zest and green beans.

- Cook and mix for 10 minutes, or till beans are soft, yet a bit crunchy.

Nutrition Information

- Calories: 106 calories;

- Total Fat: 9.7

- Sodium: 106

- Total Carbohydrate: 4.8

- Cholesterol: 8

- Protein: 1.1

Fried Squash Blossoms

Serving: 4

Ingredients

- 12 zucchini blossoms

- 2 eggs, beaten

- 1/2 cup all-purpose flour

- 1/2 cup Italian bread crumbs

- 2 tablespoons olive oil

- salt and ground black pepper, to taste

Direction

- Slowly dunk zucchini blossoms in beaten egg and shake excess off. Pat into the flour; cover with bread crumbs. On a plate, put the breaded blossoms; avoid stacking.

- In a big frying pan, heat olive oil over medium-high heat. In batches, fry blossoms for about 5 minutes per side till each side are golden brown. Put black pepper and salt to season.

Nutrition Information

Calories: 211 calories;

Total Fat: 10.2

Sodium: 300

Total Carbohydrate: 22.6

Cholesterol: 93

Protein: 6.9

Gandule Rice

Serving: 20

Ingredients

1 cup vegetable oil

3 pounds pork shoulder, cubed

3 tablespoons achiote (annatto) seeds

2 cups chopped onion

2 cups chopped fresh cilantro

12 cloves garlic, crushed

2 tablespoons salt

1 teaspoon ground black pepper

2 (8 ounce) cans tomato sauce

1 (15 ounce) can pigeon peas, drained

15 ounces black olives, pitted and halved

8 cups uncooked calrose rice, rinsed

9 cups water

Direction

In a big saucepan set on medium-high heat, add 2 tablespoons of the oil. Put in pork and brown in oil. In the meantime, put the rest of the oil in a small saucepan set on medium heat then place in achiote seeds. Then heat until the oil turns a dark orange or red. Separate from heat and reserve.

Add pepper, salt, garlic, cilantro, and onion to the ground pork. Then cook to shrink veggies, and mix in olives, pigeon peas, and tomato sauce. Stir well. Drain achiote/oil mixture to the pork mixture and mix well. Lower heat and allow it to simmer for 10 minutes.

Mix water and uncooked rice to pork mixture; mix thoroughly. Bring temperature to high, then cover the saucepan and make it boil. Whisk again, lower heat then cover; allow it to cook on low for approximately 10 minutes. Uncover, mix again, put the cover back and cook for 10 more minutes; mix again. Separate from heat and let it rest for 15 minutes.

Nutrition Information

Calories: 615 calories;

Protein: 18.6

Total Fat: 27.6

Sodium: 1112

Total Carbohydrate: 71.7

Cholesterol: 48

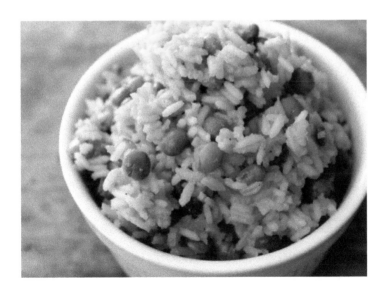

Garlic Asparagus With Lime

Serving: 4

Ingredients

1 teaspoon butter

1 tablespoon olive oil

1 clove garlic, minced

1 medium shallot, minced

1 bunch fresh asparagus spears, trimmed

1/4 lime, juiced

salt and pepper to taste

Direction

Place the large skillet over medium heat. Melt the butter with olive oil into the hot skillet. Stir in shallots and garlic and let it cook for 1-2 minutes. Mix in asparagus spears and cook for 5 minutes until tender. Pour the squeezed

lime over the mixture. Season it with salt and pepper.
Serve it on a serving plate together with lime wedges for
garnish.

Nutrition Information

Calories: 73 calories;

Sodium: 11

Total Carbohydrate: 7.2

Cholesterol: 3

Protein: 2.9

Total Fat: 4.5

Garlic Potatoes Gratin

Serving: 8

Ingredients

3 pounds red potatoes, peeled and sliced

6 ounces Gouda cheese, shredded, divided

3 tablespoons butter

5 cloves garlic, minced

1 1/2 cups heavy cream

1 teaspoon salt

1/2 teaspoon black pepper

Direction

Preheat the oven to 165°C or 325°F. Lightly oil a baking dish, 9x13 inch in size.

Layer half of potatoes, half the cheese, then the rest of the potatoes in the prepped dish.

In a small skillet, liquify butter over medium heat. Sauté garlic till golden brown and aromatic; put on top of potatoes.

Mix pepper, salt and cream; put equally on top of potatoes and scatter the rest of the cheese over.

In prepped oven, let bake for 75 minutes. Serve right away.

Nutrition Information

Calories: 394 calories;

Sodium: 524

Total Carbohydrate: 29.5

Cholesterol: 97

Protein: 9.6

Total Fat: 26.9

Garlic Red Potatoes

Serving: 4

Ingredients

- 2 pounds red potatoes, quartered

- 1/4 cup butter, melted

- 2 teaspoons minced garlic

- 1 teaspoon salt

- 1 lemon, juiced

- 1 tablespoon grated Parmesan cheese

Direction

Heat the oven to 350 degrees Fahrenheit or 175 degrees Celsius.

Place the potatoes in a baking dish (8x8 inches).

In a small bowl, combine the lemon juice, salt, garlic, and melted butter, then pour over the potatoes, stirring to coat. Sprinkle with Parmesan cheese.

Bake while covered in the preheated oven for 30 minutes. Uncover, and bake for another 10 minutes until potatoes are soft when pierced using a fork, and golden brown.

Nutrition Information

Calories: 279 calories;

Total Fat: 12.2

Sodium: 698

Total Carbohydrate: 39.6

Cholesterol: 32

Protein: 5.3

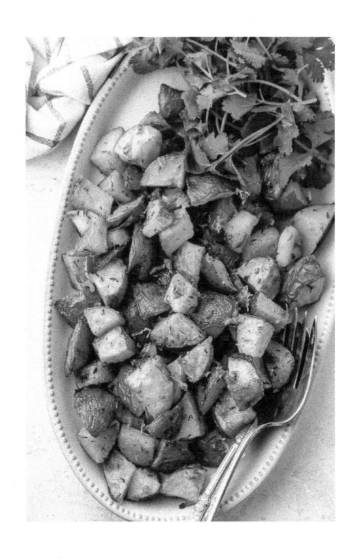

Garlicky Summer Squash And Fresh Corn

Serving: 6

Ingredients

- 2 tablespoons olive oil

- 1/2 yellow onion, sliced

- 4 cloves garlic, minced

- 1/2 cup vegetable broth

- 1 ear corn, kernels cut from cob

- 2 cups sliced yellow squash

- 2 cups sliced zucchini

- 1 tablespoon chopped fresh parsley

- 2 tablespoons butter

- salt and pepper to taste

Direction

- In a skillet, heat oil over medium-high heat, and let garlic and onion cook till slightly soft. Add in corn kernels and vegetable broth, and allow to cook till heated through. Add in zucchini and squash. Put a cover, and keep cooking for 10 minutes, mixing from time to time, till zucchini and squash are soft.

- Into the skillet with squash, put butter and parsley. Put pepper and salt to season. Allow to cook and mix till the butter is liquefied, and serve while hot.

Nutrition Information

- Calories: 111 calories;

- Total Carbohydrate: 8

- Cholesterol: 10

- Protein: 1.8

- Total Fat: 8.8

- Sodium: 74

Georgian Green Beans

Serving: 10

Ingredients

- 2 pounds fresh green beans, trimmed

- 3 tablespoons unsalted butter

- 1 large red onion, quartered and thinly sliced

- 2 cloves garlic, peeled and minced

- 1 1/2 teaspoons red wine vinegar

- 3 tablespoons chicken broth

- salt and pepper to taste

- 3 tablespoons finely chopped cilantro

Direction

- Boil a big pot of lightly salted water. Put green beans in the water and cook for 3 minutes. Take off from heat, drain in a colander. Put under cold water until it's not hot. Drain then pat dry.

- In a medium skillet, melt 1 tbsp. butter on medium heat. Mix in garlic and onion. Sauté until onions are tender. Melt leftover butter in skillet. Mix green beans in. Mix in broth and vinegar. Season with pepper and salt. Stir in cilantro. Lower heat, simmer, covered, for 15 minutes or until the green beans are tender.

Nutrition Information

- Calories: 66 calories;
- Sodium: 7
- Total Carbohydrate: 8.2
- Cholesterol: 9
- Protein: 1.9
- Total Fat: 3.6

Gnocchi In Fontina Sauce

Serving: 4

Ingredients

- 1 pound refrigerated gnocchi

- 6 tablespoons unsalted butter

- 2 tablespoons chopped shallots

- 8 ounces Italian fontina cheese, cubed

- 1/3 cup heavy cream

- 3 tablespoons freshly grated Parmesan cheese

- 1 tablespoon chopped fresh basil

Direction

- Boil a big pot of slightly salted water. Put gnocchi, and allow to cook for 5 minutes till soft. Let drain, and reserve.

- Meanwhile, prepare the sauce, as you desire gnocchi to finish first. In a saucepan, liquify the butter over medium heat. Put shallots, and allow to cook for several minutes, till soft. Mix in cream, and heat to nearly a boil. Slowly add in parmesan and fontina cheeses, prevent from boiling. Mix till smooth, then take off from the heat quickly, or the sauce will clump.

- Into serving dishes, put the gnocchi, and scoop sauce on top of each. Jazz up with chopped fresh basil.

Nutrition Information

- Calories: 624 calories;

- Total Fat: 51.3

- Sodium: 607

- Total Carbohydrate: 22.5

- Cholesterol: 163

- Protein: 19.6

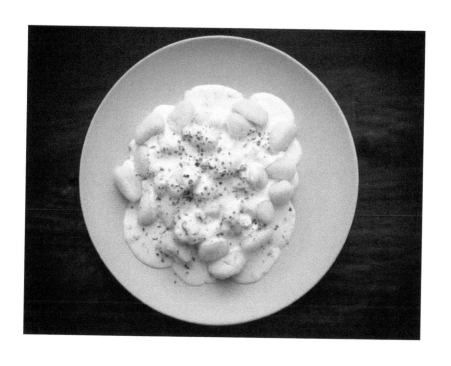

Gobi Aloo (Indian Style Cauliflower With Potatoes)

Serving: 4

Ingredients

- 1 tablespoon vegetable oil

- 1 teaspoon cumin seeds

- 1 teaspoon minced garlic

- 1 teaspoon ginger paste

- 2 medium potatoes, peeled and cubed

- 1/2 teaspoon ground turmeric

- 1/2 teaspoon paprika

- 1 teaspoon ground cumin

- 1/2 teaspoon garam masala

- salt to taste

- 1 pound cauliflower

- 1 teaspoon chopped fresh cilantro

Direction

- In a medium skillet, heat oil over medium heat. Mix in ginger paste, garlic and cumin seeds. Let cook till garlic is lightly browned, for about a minute. Place in potatoes. Put salt, garam masala, cumin, paprika and turmeric to season. Cover and keep cooking for 5 to 7 minutes, mixing from time to time.

- Into the saucepan, combine the cilantro and cauliflower. Lower heat to low and put cover. Mixing from time to time, keep cooking for 10 minutes, or till cauliflower and potatoes are soft.

Nutrition Information

- Calories: 135 calories;

- Sodium: 331

- Total Carbohydrate: 23.1

- Cholesterol: 0

- Protein: 4

- Total Fat: 4

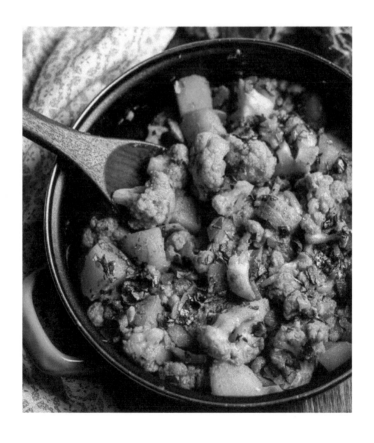

Grandma's Artichokes

Serving: 4

Ingredients

- 4 whole artichokes, trimmed and coarse outer leaves removed

- 8 large cloves garlic, chopped

- 1 tablespoon salt, or to taste

- 1 tablespoon ground black pepper

- 1/4 cup grated Romano cheese

- 1 bunch flat-leaf parsley, leaves torn

- 1/2 cup peanut oil

Direction

- Clip stems of artichoke flat to make artichokes stand upright and wash well under running water. On a work surface, hold the artichokes upside down and open the leaves by lightly smashing the artichokes. Scatter a quarter of the garlic into the spaces between the leaves of every artichoke.

- Put black pepper, salt to season the artichokes and a tablespoon of grated Romano cheese for each artichoke, exposing the leaves and allowing the cheese and seasonings into the leaves. Into spaces among the leaves, force torn leaves of parsley to keep the seasonings in.

- In a saucepan, place the artichokes upright and put peanut oil on top, allowing the oil to seep into openings between the leaves. Into the saucepan, carefully put water, keep water from splashing on artichokes and wash off the oil. Cover the pan.

- Boil, turn the heat to low, and gently simmer for an hour till the outer leaves of the artichoke are easy to take off yet not falling apart or mushy. Adjust the taste by putting additional salt if wished; allow to simmer for 5 to 10 minutes longer to let the salt melt.

Nutrition Information

Calories: 352 calories;

Total Fat: 29.4

Sodium: 1964

Total Carbohydrate: 19

Cholesterol: 8

Protein: 7.8

Greek Potato Stew

Serving: 6

Ingredients

- 2 1/2 pounds potatoes, peeled and cubed
- 1/3 cup olive oil
- 2 cloves garlic, minced
- 3/4 cup whole, pitted kalamata olives
- 1 1/3 cups chopped tomatoes
- 1 teaspoon dried oregano
- salt and pepper to taste

Direction

- Heat the oil in a big sauté pan over medium heat. Put in the potatoes then stir. Mix in garlic then put in the olives and cook and stir for several minutes. Mix in oregano and tomatoes.

- Decrease the heat then cover. Allow to simmer until potatoes become tender, about 30 minutes. Use pepper and salt to season.

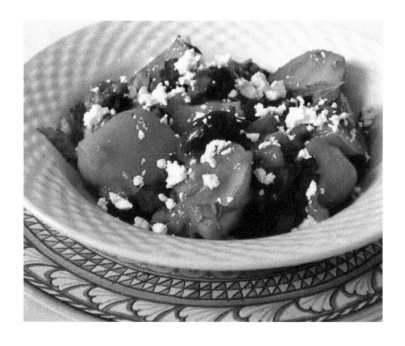

Green Beans With Orange Olive Oil

Serving: 4

Ingredients

- 3/4 pound fresh green beans, trimmed and halved

- 4 1/2 teaspoons extra-virgin olive oil

- 1 tablespoon orange zest strips

- kosher salt to taste

- 1 teaspoon grated orange zest

Direction

- In a steamer basket on top of an inch boiling water, put the green beans and cover. Let cook for 2 to 4 minutes till beans are soft yet remain firm. Drain; retain warmth.

- In the meantime, in a large skillet, mix together 1 tablespoon orange zest strips and olive oil over medium-low heat. Let cook and mix for about 2 minutes till olive oil has been infused with flavor of orange zest. Get rid of zest strips.

- With flavored olive oil and kosher salt, toss the drained green beans over medium heat till beans are covered in oil and hot. Put onto a serving platter and garnish with leftover 1 teaspoon grated orange zest.

Nutrition Information

Calories: 76 calories;

Cholesterol: 0

Protein: 1.6

Total Fat: 5.4

Sodium: 105

Total Carbohydrate: 6.6

Grilled Beets In Rosemary Vinegar

Serving: 6

Ingredients

- 1/3 cup balsamic vinegar

- 1 teaspoon chopped fresh rosemary

- 1 clove garlic, peeled and crushed

- 1/2 teaspoon herbes de Provence

- 3 medium beets, sliced into rounds

Direction

- Mix herbes de Provence, garlic, rosemary and balsamic vinegar in a medium bowl. Add beets in the mixture. Marinate for 20 minutes minimum.

- Preheat outdoor grill to high heat; oil the grate lightly.

- On a piece of foil, big enough to wrap all the ingredients, put the marinated mixture and beets; tightly seal. Put foil packet on the prepared grill. Cook till beets are tender for 25 minutes.

- Take beets out of the packet. Put it on the grill grate directly for 2-5 minutes. Serve while hot.

Nutrition Information

- Calories: 27 calories;

- Protein: 0.7

- Total Fat: 0.1

- Sodium: 36

- Total Carbohydrate: 6.2

- Cholesterol: 0

Grilled Portobellos Sauteed In Wine

Serving: 4

Ingredients

- 4 portobello mushroom caps

- 1 tablespoon olive oil

- 1 tablespoon butter

- 1 shallot, thinly sliced

- 1 cup white wine

Direction

- Start by preheating the grill to high heat.

- Onto the grill, put the mushrooms with the smooth side turning up. Grill for about 10 minutes until they begin to get tender. Flip over, and grill the other side, about 5 minutes.

- In the meantime, in a big frying pan, heat butter and olive oil over medium heat. Put in shallot and fry for several minutes, tossing often.

- Transfer the mushrooms onto a cutting board and cut. Add to the frying pan, and raise the heat to high. Cook for 1 minute, and then add wine. Keep stirring and cooking until the wine has almost evaporated. Take away from heat and enjoy.

Nutrition Information

- Calories: 145 calories;
- Total Fat: 6.5
- Sodium: 32
- Total Carbohydrate: 9.4
- Cholesterol: 8
- Protein: 3.2

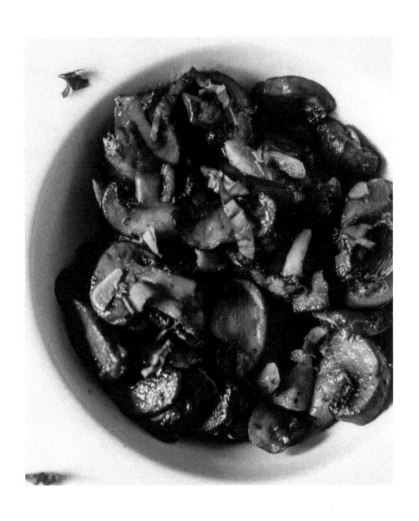

Grilled Tequila Cilantro Pineapple

Serving: 4

Ingredients

- 1 fresh pineapple, peeled and cored

- 1 cup chopped fresh cilantro

- 1 cup tequila

- 1 1/2 tablespoons ground chipotle chiles

- 1 lemon

- 1 lime

- salt and pepper to taste

Direction

- Lengthwise, cut pineapple to 8 wedges. Put wedges into sealable plastic bag/container. Mix chipotle, tequila and cilantro in a small bowl. Put into container with pineapple. Cut lime and lemon in half. Squeeze some juice out; put fruit and juice into container. Season with pepper and salt. Marinate for 1 hour minimum in the fridge, flipping pineapple once.

- Preheat outdoor grill for medium high heat. Brush a light coat of oil on grate when coals are hot.

- Grill wedges, 4-5 minutes per side. For sauce: Cook marinade on medium high heat in a saucepan; boil. Cook till sauce is syrupy and thick. It will be spicy.

Nutrition Information

- Calories: 206 calories;

- Total Fat: 0.4

- Sodium: 34

- Total Carbohydrate: 20.9

- Cholesterol: 0

- Protein: 1.3

Guinean Peanut Sauce With Butternut Squash

Serving: 4

Ingredients

- 1 butternut squash - peeled, seeded, and cut into 2-inch cubes

- 1/2 cup natural peanut butter

- 1 small tomato, chopped

- 1 cup warm water

- 2 tablespoons olive oil

- 1 large yellow onion, thickly sliced lengthwise

- 2 cloves garlic, minced

- 1 bay leaf

- ground black pepper to taste

- salt, or to taste

- 2 teaspoons lemon juice

Direction

- In a saucepan, put butternut squash with enough water to cover. Boil and simmer with a cover for 20 minutes, till squash is soft. Drain, setting aside the cooking liquid.

- In a bowl, mix together warm water, tomato and peanut butter. Squish it together by hand or use a food processor.

- In a skillet over medium-high heat, heat the olive oil. Once oil is hot, put in slices of onion and cook for 2 minutes. Put in about 1/2 teaspoon salt, black pepper, bay leaf, minced garlic and peanut butter mixture. Mix to incorporate, then boil.

- Turn heat down to low and let the peanut sauce simmer for 15 minutes, putting in the reserved cooking liquid as necessary. The consistency should resemble a thick soup.

- Mix in butternut squash and simmer for 15 minutes more. Put in lemon juice, and taste to alter seasoning.

Nutrition Information

- Calories: 396 calories;

- Protein: 11.4

- Total Fat: 24

- Sodium: 391

- Total Carbohydrate: 42.4

- Cholesterol: 0

Haricots Verts Lyonnaise

Serving: 4

Ingredients

16 cups water

1 tablespoon sea salt

1 1/2 pounds fresh green beans, rinsed and trimmed

3 tablespoons unsalted butter

1 clove garlic, crushed

1 large red onion, sliced in rings

1 pinch dried thyme

2 tablespoons red wine vinegar

sea salt to taste

ground black pepper to taste

freshly ground nutmeg to taste

1 tablespoon finely minced fresh parsley

Direction

Boil salted water in a big pot. Into the boiling water, cautiously drop green beans, by handfuls. Bring water back to a boil for 5 minutes. Drain beans right away; for 5 minutes, dunk them into ice water. Let to drain and wrap using a clean cloth; reserve.

Heat butter using the same pot over medium heat. Brown the garlic lightly. Take off from heat and put aside for 20 minutes.

Take the garlic off from butter and throw it away. Put thyme and onions to garlic flavored butter. Cover pot and braise onion for 5 minutes over medium heat, or till transparent and tender. Turn heat to medium-high, remove pot's cover and caramelize the onion lightly.

Into the pot, mix the green beans. 1 to 2 minutes later, using red wine vinegar, de glaze the pot. Season with nutmeg, pepper and sea salt to taste. Drizzle parsley on top.

Nutrition Information

Calories: 148 calories;

Sodium: 1334

Total Carbohydrate: 16.7

Cholesterol: 23

Protein: 3.7

Total Fat: 8.9

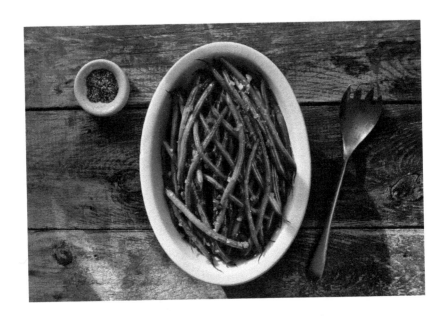

Hearts Of Palm Risotto

Serving: 2

Ingredients

1 tablespoon butter

1 tablespoon olive oil

1/2 cup finely chopped onion

2/3 cup Arborio rice

1/4 cup dry white wine

3 cups boiling vegetable broth

1/2 cup sliced hearts of palm

1/4 cup grated Parmesan cheese

salt and pepper to taste

1 tablespoon chopped fresh parsley

1 tablespoon butter

Direction

Take a big and heavy pot and heat a tablespoon of butter and olive oil on medium high heat. Add onion and cook for 2 minutes, while stirring, until edges start to turn golden brown. Put in rice and cook for 2-3 minutes until it is coated with oil and starts to toast. Lower to medium heat and add white wine. Cook until white wine has almost completely evaporated; then add 1/3 of boiling vegetable broth. Stir until blended. Repeat process 2 more times while stirring constantly. It takes 15-20 minutes to get all the broth integrated.

Once rice almost completely soft but is still a little crunchy, mix in parmesan and hearts of palm. Sprinkle with salt and pepper to season. Cook for 1 minute then mix in butter and parsley. Serve right away.

Nutrition Information

Calories: 573 calories;

Cholesterol: 39

Protein: 12

Total Fat: 22.2

Sodium: 1085

Total Carbohydrate: 75.2

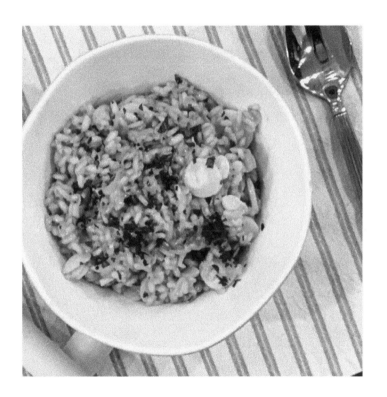

Honey Roasted Red Potatoes

Serving: 4

Ingredients

1 pound red potatoes, quartered

2 tablespoons diced onion

2 tablespoons butter, melted

1 tablespoon honey

1 teaspoon dry mustard

1 pinch salt

1 pinch ground black pepper

Direction

Preheat the oven to 190°C or 375°F. With nonstick cooking spray, lightly coat an 11x7-inch baking dish.

In prepped dish, put potatoes in 1 layer; place onion on top. Mix pepper, salt, mustard, honey and melted butter in a small bowl; sprinkle on top of potatoes and onion.

In the preheated 190°C or 375°F oven, let to bake for 35 minutes or till soft, mixing halfway through cooking time.

Nutrition Information

Calories: 156 calories;

Total Fat: 6.2

Sodium: 88

Total Carbohydrate: 23.4

Cholesterol: 15

Protein: 2.5

Honey And Rosemary Sweet Potatoes

Serving: 6

Ingredients

- 2 tablespoons olive oil

- 1/4 cup honey

- 2 tablespoons chopped fresh rosemary

- 1 teaspoon salt

- 1 teaspoon freshly ground black pepper

- 3 large sweet potatoes, peeled and cut in 1-inch cubes

Direction

Heat the oven beforehand to 175 °C or 350 °F. Line parchment paper or foil on a baking sheet.

In a big bowl, combine black pepper, salt, rosemary, honey and olive oil together. Coat the sweet potato cubes by stirring them in the mixture in the bowl. Use slotted spoon to remove sweet potato cubes from the mixture. Spread the coated sweet potato cubes on the prepared baking sheet in a single layer.

Bake for about 45 minutes in the preheated oven until tender. Turn the oven temperature to 230 °C or 450 °F. Bake for 15 minutes more until brown.

Nutrition Information

Calories: 280 calories;

Total Fat: 4.7

Sodium: 513

Total Carbohydrate: 57.7

Cholesterol: 0

Protein: 3.7

Horseradish Beets (Chrin)

Serving: 10

Ingredients

8 (15 ounce) cans canned beets

2 (4 ounce) jars prepared horseradish

Direction

Grind the beets in an electric blender, then drain (reserve the juice for soup if desired).

Stir in the horseradish into the beets and stir well. Let it chill in the fridge until serving time.

Nutrition Information

Calories: 84 calories;

Sodium: 527

Total Carbohydrate: 19.5

Cholesterol: 0

Protein: 2.4

Total Fat: 0.5

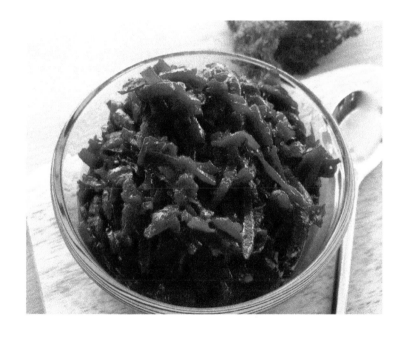

Quick And Easy Squash Blossoms

Serving: 2

Ingredients

1 tablespoon butter

6 yellow squash blossoms

4 fresh basil leaves, chopped

4 fresh oregano leaves, chopped

4 fresh thyme leaves, chopped

1 clove garlic, minced

2 tablespoons white wine

6 ounces green chile sauce (such as Coyote Trail®)

Direction

In a big skillet, melt butter over medium heat. Put garlic, thyme, oregano, basil and squash; cook and mix for about a minute till aromatic. Put in wine; let cook for a minute longer.

Take off skillet from heat and mix in the green chili sauce. Allow to stand, with cover, for about 5 minutes till flavors incorporate.

Nutrition Information

- Calories: 100 calories;
- Cholesterol: 15
- Protein: 3.5
- Total Fat: 6.7
- Sodium: 2266
- Total Carbohydrate: 5.7

Indian Cabbage Patties

Serving: 20

Ingredients

2 dried red chiles, stemmed and seeded

1 cup fresh grated coconut

1 cup rice flour

1/2 cup gram flour (chickpea flour)

1 tablespoon tamarind, or as needed

4 tablespoons coriander seeds

1 tablespoon skinned split black lentils (urad dal)

1 tablespoon asafoetida powder

1 medium head cabbage, shredded

1 pinch salt to taste

1 pinch white sugar, or to taste

oil for frying

Direction

On medium-high heat, heat a heavy pan. Toast chiles in the pan for 2-4 minutes, turning often, until fragrant, until fragrant. Put toasted chiles in a blender.

In the blender with chiles, process tamarind, gram flour, rice flour and coconut to make a fine paste. Put a bit of water if needed.

In a skillet, heat 2 tbsp. oil on high heat. Stir and cook asafoetida, urad dal and coriander for 30 seconds. Put this in the blender with tamarind mixture. Blend to incorporate.

In a big bowl, put shredded cabbage and coriander-tamarind paste. Mix to combine. Season using sugar and salt.

In a heavy, big skillet, heat oil to fry. Spread small cabbage mixture portions in hot pan. Fry patties for 2-3 minutes per side until brown.

Nutrition Information

Calories: 126 calories;

Total Carbohydrate: 13.1

Cholesterol: 0

Protein: 2.2

Total Fat: 7.9

Sodium: 19

Indian Style Basmati Rice

Serving: 6

Ingredients

1 1/2 cups basmati rice

2 tablespoons vegetable oil

1 (2 inch) piece cinnamon stick

2 pods green cardamom

2 whole cloves

1 tablespoon cumin seed

1 teaspoon salt, or to taste

2 1/2 cups water

1 small onion, thinly sliced

Direction

- Into a bowl, put rice with sufficient water to submerge. Reserve for 20 minutes to soak.

- In a saucepan or big pot, heat oil over medium heat.

- Put cumin seed, cloves, cardamom pods and cinnamon stick. Let cook and mix for approximately 1 minute, then to the pot, put the onion.

- Sauté for 10 minutes till onion is rich golden brown in color. Strain the water from the rice, and mix into the pot.

- Let cook and mix the rice for several minutes, till slightly toasted. To the pot, put water and salt, and boil.

- Put a cover, and turn the heat to low. Let simmer for approximately 15 minutes, or till all the water has been soaked in.

- Let sit for 5 minutes, then fluff using a fork prior to serving.

Nutrition Information

Calories: 216 calories;

Sodium: 394

Total Carbohydrate: 38.9

Cholesterol: 0

Protein: 3.9

Total Fat: 5.4

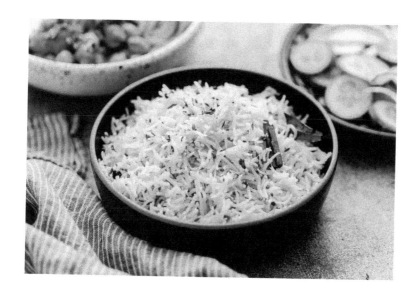

Jasmine's Brussels Sprouts

Serving: 4

Ingredients

- 3 cups water

- 1 pound Brussels sprouts, trimmed

- 2 tablespoons olive oil

- 2 cloves garlic, minced

- 8 ounces pancetta bacon, diced

- 1 teaspoon salt

- 1 teaspoon ground black pepper

Direction

- Fill a big saucepan with water and lead it to boiling point.

- Insert the Brussels sprouts and leaving it cooking for 5-7 minutes.

- By the end, the sprouts should maintain a slight firmness to it. After draining the sprouts, run them through cold water and halve the sprouts up by slicing.

- Put them to one side. Pour in 1-tablespoon olive oil into a big skillet and warm it up at medium high heat.

- Insert the pancetta and garlic, cooking and stirring until the garlic starts browning a little, around 5 minutes.

- Insert Brussels sprouts and the rest of the olive oil.

- Lower the heat setting to medium then continue cooking. Stir until the sprouts are thoroughly flavored.

- Add pepper and salt, cooking for another 5 minutes.

- Serve.

Nutrition Information

- Calories: 369 calories;

- Total Fat: 32.3

- Sodium: 1077

- Total Carbohydrate: 11.4

- Cholesterol: 38

- Protein: 10.5

Kaese Spaetzle

Serving: 8

Ingredients

- 1 1/2 cups all-purpose flour

- 3/4 teaspoon ground nutmeg

- 3/4 teaspoon salt

- 1/8 teaspoon pepper

- 3 eggs

- 3/8 cup 2% milk

- 3 tablespoons butter

- 1 onion, sliced

- 1 1/2 cups shredded Emmentaler cheese

Direction

- Sift together pepper, salt, nutmeg and flour. In a medium bowl, whisk the eggs. Alternately stir in milk and flour mixture till smooth. Let sit for half an hour.

- Boil a big pot of slightly salted water. Press batter through a spaetzle press into the water. Alternatively, use a cheese grater, colander or a potato ricer. Once spaetzle has risen to surface of the water, transfer it to a bowl using a slotted spoon. Stir in a cup of cheese.

- In a big skillet, melt butter over medium-high heat. Put in onion, and cook till golden. Mix in the rest of the cheese and the spaetzle till well incorporated. Take away from heat, and serve right away.

Nutrition Information

Calories: 245 calories;

Cholesterol: 102

Protein: 11.5

Total Fat: 13.1

Sodium: 377

Total Carbohydrate: 20.1

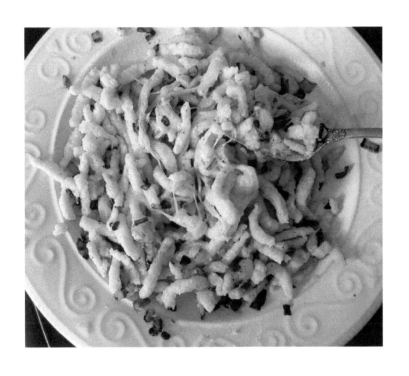

Kartoshnik With Cheese And Onions

Serving: 11

Ingredients

- 3 large potatoes, peeled and quartered

- 5 eggs

- 1/4 cup heavy whipping cream

- 3/4 teaspoon salt

- 3/4 cup shredded sharp Cheddar cheese

- 3/4 cup shredded Swiss cheese

- 1/2 onion, chopped

- 3 teaspoons baking powder

- 1/2 cup butter, melted

- 1/2 cup sour cream

- 1/2 cup chopped green onions

Direction

- Put potatoes in a medium pot, submerge in water and let boil till cooked. Once done, drain the water and throw. Crush potatoes and reserve.

- Preheat the oven to 230°C or 450°F. With a no-stick vegetable spray, coat a 9x9-inch oven-proof baking dish or massage inner with margarine or butter.

- Whisk eggs in another bowl, put salt and whipping cream, and beat till incorporated. Put crushed potatoes and combine till well incorporated. Put onions and both cheeses and mix thoroughly. Put baking powder and combine well. Into prepped baking dish, put the potato mixture and level.

- Bake at for 35 minutes in the preheated oven or till top is light brown. Take off from the oven and allow to cool for 5 minutes. When cooking, Kartoshnik will rise, yet will subside once taken off from the oven and lightly cooled.

- Liquify margarine or butter in a small pot.

- Into 3x3-inch squares, slice Kartoshnik and serve together with liquified margarine or butter, a dollop of sour cream, and a sprinkling of green onions. You may use low fat sour cream or plain yogurt if desired.

Nutrition Information

- Calories: 295 calories;

- Total Fat: 20.1

- Sodium: 470

- Total Carbohydrate: 20

- Cholesterol: 135

- Protein: 9.9

Kathy's Baked Stuffed Tomatoes

Serving: 4

Ingredients

- 1 (15 ounce) can garbanzo beans

- 4 ounces trimmed arugula

- 1 tablespoon minced garlic

- 1/4 cup crumbled feta cheese

- 5 tablespoons grated Parmesan cheese, divided

- 1/4 cup olive oil

- 4 tomatoes, tops and pulp removed

Direction

- Set the oven to 375°F or 190°C for preheating.

- Blend the arugula, feta cheese, olive oil, garbanzo beans, 4 tbsp. of Parmesan cheese, and garlic in a food processor or blender until smooth.

- In an 8x8-inches baking dish, arrange the tomatoes and stuff them with the garbanzo bean mixture. Sprinkle it with the remaining Parmesan dish.

- Let it bake inside the preheated oven for 20 minutes until lightly browned and bubbly.

Nutrition Information

Calories: 303 calories;

Total Fat: 19.9

Sodium: 495

Total Carbohydrate: 23.3

Cholesterol: 20

Protein: 10

Kreplach

Serving: 8

Ingredients

- 4 tablespoons vegetable oil

- 2 pounds lean ground beef

- 4 onions, chopped

- salt and pepper to taste

- 1 pinch ground cinnamon (optional)

- 1/8 cup crushed walnuts

- 2 cups all-purpose flour

- 1/2 teaspoon salt

- 2 eggs

- 1 1/2 cups warm water

Direction

- Heat oil in a big skillet over medium heat and put nuts, cinnamon, salt and pepper to taste, onions and beef; cook till beef is not pink anymore. Take off from heat and allow to cool.

- Mix water, eggs, salt and flour in a big mixing bowl; combine till dough is smooth. Form dough into a round and split into 10 portions.

- Roll flat every portion of dough on a floured board; cut out 5 circles, approximately 3 inches in diameter. In the center of every circle, put about a teaspoon of meat filling; fold dough over and secure edges with a little amount of water.

- Boil a big pot of lightly salted water; drop in the kreplach, several at a time. Let cook for 4 minutes or till kreplach rises on the surface. Take off using a slotted spoon; serve.

Nutrition Information

- Calories: 527 calories;

- Total Fat: 33.2

- Sodium: 244

- Total Carbohydrate: 29.4

- Cholesterol: 132

- Protein: 25.8

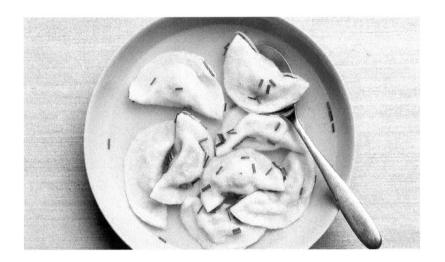

Lemon Green Beans With Walnuts

Serving: 4

Ingredients

- 1/2 cup chopped walnuts

- 1 pound green beans, trimmed and cut into 2 inch pieces

- 2 1/2 tablespoons unsalted butter, melted

- 1 lemon, juiced and zested

- salt and pepper to taste

Direction

- Preheat the oven to 190 °C or 375 °F. On a baking sheet, set nuts in 1 layer. In the prepped oven, toast till slightly browned, about 5 to 10 minutes.

- In a steamer over of 1 inch of boiling water, put the green beans, and cover. Steam for 8 to 10 minutes, or till soft, yet bright green.

- In a big bowl, put the cooked beans, and toss together with lemon zest, lemon juice and butter. Put in pepper and salt to season. On a serving dish, place the beans, and scatter toasted walnuts on top. Serve right away.

Nutrition Information

- Calories: 202 calories;

- Cholesterol: 19

- Protein: 4.7

- Total Fat: 17.2

- Sodium: 9

- Total Carbohydrate: 13

Mangu

Serving: 6

Ingredients

- 3 green plantains

- 1 quart water

- 1/4 cup olive oil

- 1 cup sliced white onion

- 1 1/2 tablespoons salt

- 1 cup sliced Anaheim peppers

Direction

- In a saucepan, put water and plantains. Boil, and cook for 20 minutes, till plantains are soft yet slightly firm. Drain, setting aside a cup of liquid. Allow plantains to cool, and take off skin.

- In a skillet over medium heat, heat olive oil, and sauté onion till soft.

- Mash plantains along with salt and reserved liquid in a bowl. Move to a food processor, stir in peppers, and puree. Serve pureed plantain mixture with onions on top.

Nutrition Information

- Calories: 210 calories;

- Total Fat: 9.5

- Sodium: 1756

- Total Carbohydrate: 33.3

- Cholesterol: 0

- Protein: 1.9

Maple Glazed Sweet Potatoes With Bacon And Caramelized Onions

Serving: 12

Ingredients

- 4 pounds sweet potatoes, peeled and cut in 1-inch chunks

- 2 tablespoons olive oil

- 1 teaspoon salt

- 1/2 teaspoon ground black pepper

- 5 slices smoked bacon, chopped

- 1 pound onions, thinly sliced

- 1 cup pure maple syrup

- 2 teaspoons fresh thyme

Direction

- Preheat an oven to 220 °C or 425 °F. In a big bowl, toss black pepper, salt, olive oil and sweet potato chunks. On a big rimmed baking sheet, arrange the sweet potatoes.

- In the prepped oven, roast for 40 minutes till soft and browned; mix after the initial 20 minutes.

- In a big skillet over medium heat, cook the bacon for 10 minutes till brown and crisp; put the bacon into a bowl, but retain grease in the skillet. In bacon grease, cook onions for 10 minutes till browned, mixing often. Turn heat down to low, and cook the onions for 10 to 15 minutes more till really tender, sweet and brown. Mix frequently. Blend onions with bacon in the bowl, and reserve.

- In the hot skillet, put maple syrup with thyme, and bring to a rolling boil. Boil syrup for 3 to 4 minutes till reduced by half. Put in onion-bacon mixture and roasted sweet potatoes, coat vegetables with maple glaze by mixing. Place into a serving dish.

Nutrition Information

- Calories: 287 calories;

- Total Fat: 7.7

- Sodium: 378

- Total Carbohydrate: 51.8

- Cholesterol: 8

- Protein: 4.2

Mushroom Onion Matzo Kugel

Serving: 4

Ingredients

- 3 cups matzo farfel

- 2 onions, chopped

- 1 pound mushrooms, chopped

- 2 tablespoons vegetable oil

- salt and pepper to taste

- 1 pinch garlic powder

- 1 teaspoon dried dill weed

Direction

- Preheat the oven to 175°C or 350°F. Oil a baking dish, 8x12-inch in size.

- In a colander, add farfel and put boiling water on top of it.

- Sauté mushrooms and onions with vegetable oil in a big skillet. Mix in dill, garlic powder, pepper and salt. Take off from heat; into the skillet, mix farfel.

- Allow to bake for an hour at 175°C or 350°F.

Nutrition Information

- Calories: 292 calories;

- Sodium: 8

- Total Carbohydrate: 49

- Cholesterol: 0

- Protein: 9.2

- Total Fat: 7.3

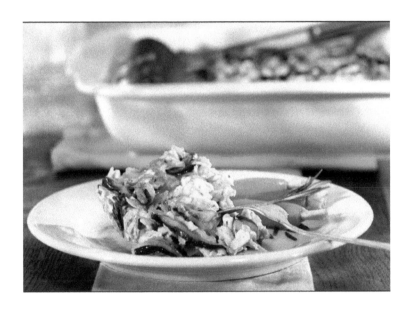

Northern Italian Cauliflower Gratin

Serving: 8

Ingredients

1 large head cauliflower, broken into florets

2 tablespoons butter

2 large cloves garlic, minced

3 tablespoons all-purpose flour

2 1/2 cups milk

1 cup heavy whipping cream

1/2 cup grated Parmesan cheese

2 ounces grated fontina cheese

1/4 teaspoon salt

1 pinch ground nutmeg

1 pinch ground white pepper

Direction

Into a saucepan, put a steamer insert and put water to just under the base of the steamer. Boil the water. Put cauliflower, cover, and let steam for 2 to 3 minutes till crisp tender. Allow to drain in a colander and quickly soak in ice water to halt the cooking process. Drain thoroughly.

Preheat the oven to 175°C or 350°F.

In a saucepan, liquify butter over low heat. Put garlic; let cook and mix for a minute till tender and aromatic. Mix in flour for 1 to 2 minutes till smooth. Put in cream and milk. Raise the heat to medium and let simmer for 5 minutes, mixing often, till sauce begins to thicken. Boil; keep cooking for 5 minutes till sauce is thick.

Into the sauce, mix white pepper, nutmeg, salt, fontina cheese and Parmesan cheese. Allow to cook for a minute, mixing forcefully, till cheese is melted into the sauce. Take off from the heat.

On the baking dish's base, scatter a cup of sauce. Set cauliflower over. Sprinkle leftover sauce on top of cauliflower, coating every floret.

In the prepped oven, bake for 10 minutes till browned lightly on top and bubbling.

Nutrition Information

Calories: 255 calories;

Total Fat: 19.2

Sodium: 301

Total Carbohydrate: 13

Cholesterol: 67

Protein: 9.4

Norwegian Potato Lefsa

Serving: 8

Ingredients

18 baking potatoes, scrubbed

1/2 cup heavy whipping cream

1/2 cup butter

1 tablespoon salt

1 tablespoon white sugar

4 cups all-purpose flour

Direction

Take skin off potatoes and put in a big pot with a generous amount of water. Boil water, and allow potatoes to boil till tender. Drain and mash thoroughly.

Mix together sugar, salt, butter, cream and 8 cups mashed potatoes in a big mixing bowl. Put a cover on bowl and chill overnight.

Stir the flour into the mashed potatoes, and roll mixture into balls, approximately the size of tennis balls, or smaller based on desire. Keep dough balls on plate in refrigerator.

Removing 1 ball from refrigerator at a time onto a floured board, roll out dough balls. Use a rolling pin with a cotton rolling pin covers to prevent dough from sticking while rolling it out.

In an iron skillet or a grill, fry lefsa at very high heat. In case lefsa brown too fast, reduce the heat. Put onto a dishtowel after cooking every piece of lefsa. Fold towel over lefsa to retain warmth. Stack lefsa on top of each other and keep covered to prevent from drying out.

Nutrition Information

Calories: 756 calories;

Sodium: 989

Total Carbohydrate: 133.4

Cholesterol: 51

Protein: 16.6

Total Fat: 18.1

Olive Oil Roasted Eggplant With Lemon

Serving: 4

Ingredients

1 large eggplant

3 tablespoons extra virgin olive oil

salt and pepper to taste

2 tablespoons fresh lemon juice

Direction

Preheat an oven to 200 °C or 400 °F. Line parchment paper on a baking sheet or oil lightly.

Halve eggplant lengthwise, then slice every half into 4 pieces lengthwise. Slice every of those in half to create 2 shorter quarters. Onto the baking sheet, put the eggplant, skin side facing down. With olive oil, brush every piece and put pepper and salt to season.

In the prepped oven; let roast for 25 minutes to half an hour till golden brown and softened. Take off from the oven and drizzle with lemon juice. Serve while hot.

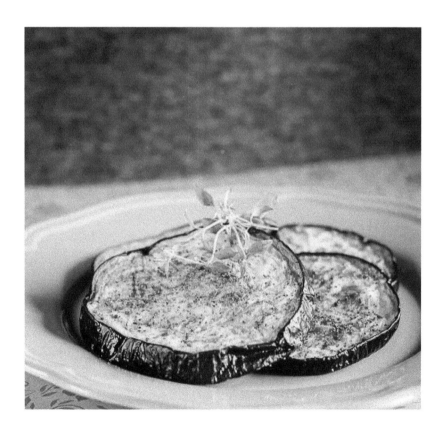

Wild Rice

Serving: 6

Ingredients

3 cups water

1 cup wild rice

1/2 teaspoon salt

1/2 cup coarsely chopped fresh morel mushrooms

1/2 cup coarsely chopped roasted chestnuts

2 green onions, chopped

6 ounces sour cream

1 green onion, chopped (optional)

salt and ground black pepper to taste

Direction

Boil 1/2 tsp. salt, wild rice and water in heavy saucepan. Lower heat to low. Cover; simmer for 30-45 minutes till wild rice is tender.

Mix 2 chopped green onions, chestnuts and morel mushrooms into rice; simmer for 15 minutes till green onions and mushrooms are tender.

Drain extra liquid; mix 1 chopped green onion and sour cream into wild rice mixture then season with black pepper and salt. Immediately serve.

Nutrition Information

Calories: 163 calories;

Total Fat: 6.5

Sodium: 216

Total Carbohydrate: 22.9

Cholesterol: 12

Protein: 4.4

Orzo Alfredo

Serving: 8

Ingredients

2 1/2 cups uncooked orzo pasta

1/4 cup unsalted butter, softened

1/4 cup heavy cream

1/4 cup grated Parmesan cheese

1 pinch nutmeg

1 tablespoon chopped fresh chives

Direction

Boil a bit pot of lightly salted water. Gradually mix in the orzo. Let the pasta cook in boiling water for 8-10 minutes or until it becomes tender; drain.

In a buttered serving bowl, put the orzo, then toss it with cream and butter and sprinkle nutmeg to season. Evenly sprinkle Parmesan cheese on top. Add chives on top to garnish.

Nutrition Information

Calories: 315 calories;

Total Fat: 10.1

Sodium: 45

Total Carbohydrate: 46.9

Cholesterol: 28

Protein: 9.7

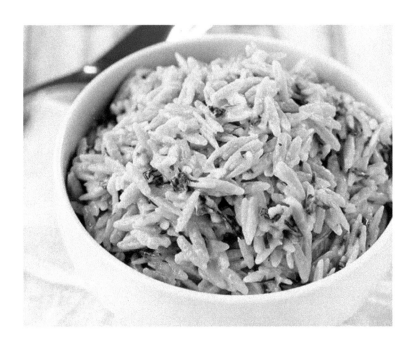

Oven Roasted Grape Tomatoes

Serving: 2

Ingredients

- 1 pound grape tomatoes, halved

- 1 tablespoon olive oil

- 2 cloves garlic, minced

- 5 fresh basil leaves, chopped

- 1 teaspoon chopped fresh thyme

- salt to taste

Direction

- Preheat the oven to 175°C or 350°F.

- In a big square of aluminum foil, put the tomatoes. Sprinkle olive oil on tomatoes and put salt, thyme, basil and garlic on top. Wrap tomato mixture with foil securing tightly to retain juices inside.

- In the preheated oven, bake for about half an hour till tomatoes are soft. Slightly cool.

Nutrition Information

- Calories: 113 calories;

- Sodium: 99

- Total Carbohydrate: 11.7

- Cholesterol: 0

- Protein: 2.2

- Total Fat: 7.5

Pakistani Spicy Chickpeas

Serving: 5

Ingredients

- 2 tablespoons vegetable oil

- 1 teaspoon cumin seeds

- 1/2 teaspoon salt

- 1/2 teaspoon chili powder

- 1/2 teaspoon lemon pepper

- 2 tomatoes, chopped

- 2 (15 ounce) cans garbanzo beans, drained

- 1 tablespoon lemon juice

- 1 onion, chopped

Direction

- Heat oil and cumin in a big pot over low heat; heat till cumin gets a darker shade of brown.

- Put in lemon and pepper seasoning, chili powder and salt; combine thoroughly. Mix in tomatoes; when juice starts to thicken, put in chickpeas and combine thoroughly.

- Put in lemon juice and combine well; put in onions and mix till tender.

- Take away from heat and put into a serving bowl; serve right away.

Nutrition Information

- Calories: 205 calories;
- Total Fat: 7.1
- Sodium: 621
- Total Carbohydrate: 30.3
- Cholesterol: 0
- Protein: 6.4

Pasta With Blue Cheese And Walnuts

Serving: 4

Ingredients

- 1/4 cup coarsely chopped walnuts

- 4 ounces blue cheese, crumbled

- 2 tablespoons olive oil

- 1/2 pound uncooked spaghetti

- 1 clove garlic, minced

Direction

- In a big pot of boiling water, cook pasta till al dente.

- In the meantime, in heavy skillet, heat the oil. Put garlic and sauté for several minutes. Mix in the walnuts; sauté for a few more minutes.

- Drain the pasta then distribute to 2 plates. Put blue cheese and sauté on top.

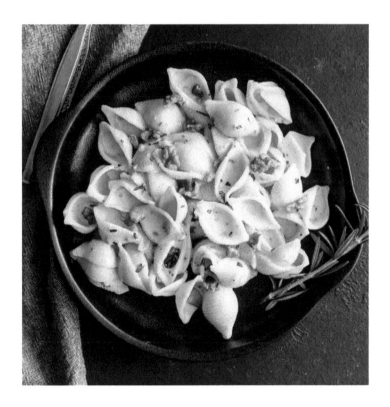

Polenta

Serving: 4

Ingredients

3 cups water

1 cup polenta

Direction

- Boil the water. Lower the heat to a simmer.

- Steadily put in polenta, mixing continuously.

- Keep on mixing till polenta is thickened. It should pull away from the sides of the pan, and able to bear a spoon. Approximately from 20 to 50 minutes.

- Onto a wooden chopping board, put the polenta, let sit for a several minutes.

Nutrition Information

- Calories: 110 calories;

- Total Fat: 1.1

- Sodium: 11

- Total Carbohydrate: 23.5

- Cholesterol: 0

- Protein: 2.5

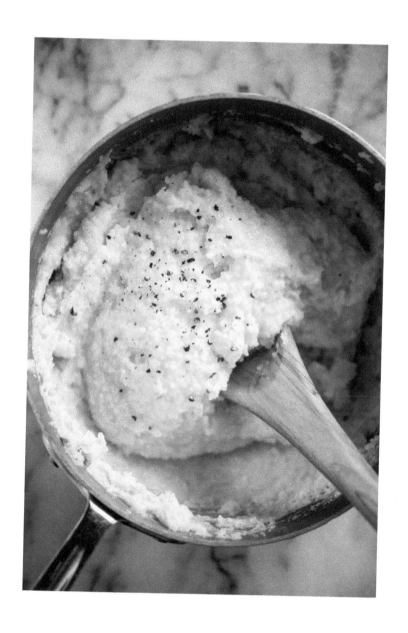

THANK YOU

Thank you for choosing *Healthy Recipes for Beginners Sides* for improving your cooking skills! I hope you enjoyed making the recipes as much as tasting them! If you're interested in learning new recipes and new meals to cook, go and check out the other books of the series.